THIS IS MY
HYSTERECTOMY
RECOVERY
COLORING
BOOK

THIS COLORING BOOK
BELONGS TO:

_____

- - - - - - - - - - - - - - - - - - -

- - - - - - - - - - - - - - - - - - -

_____

HYSTERCTOMY SURGERY

RECOVERY LOADING
PLEASE WAIT...

BET YOU ARE GLAD THAT IS OVARIES

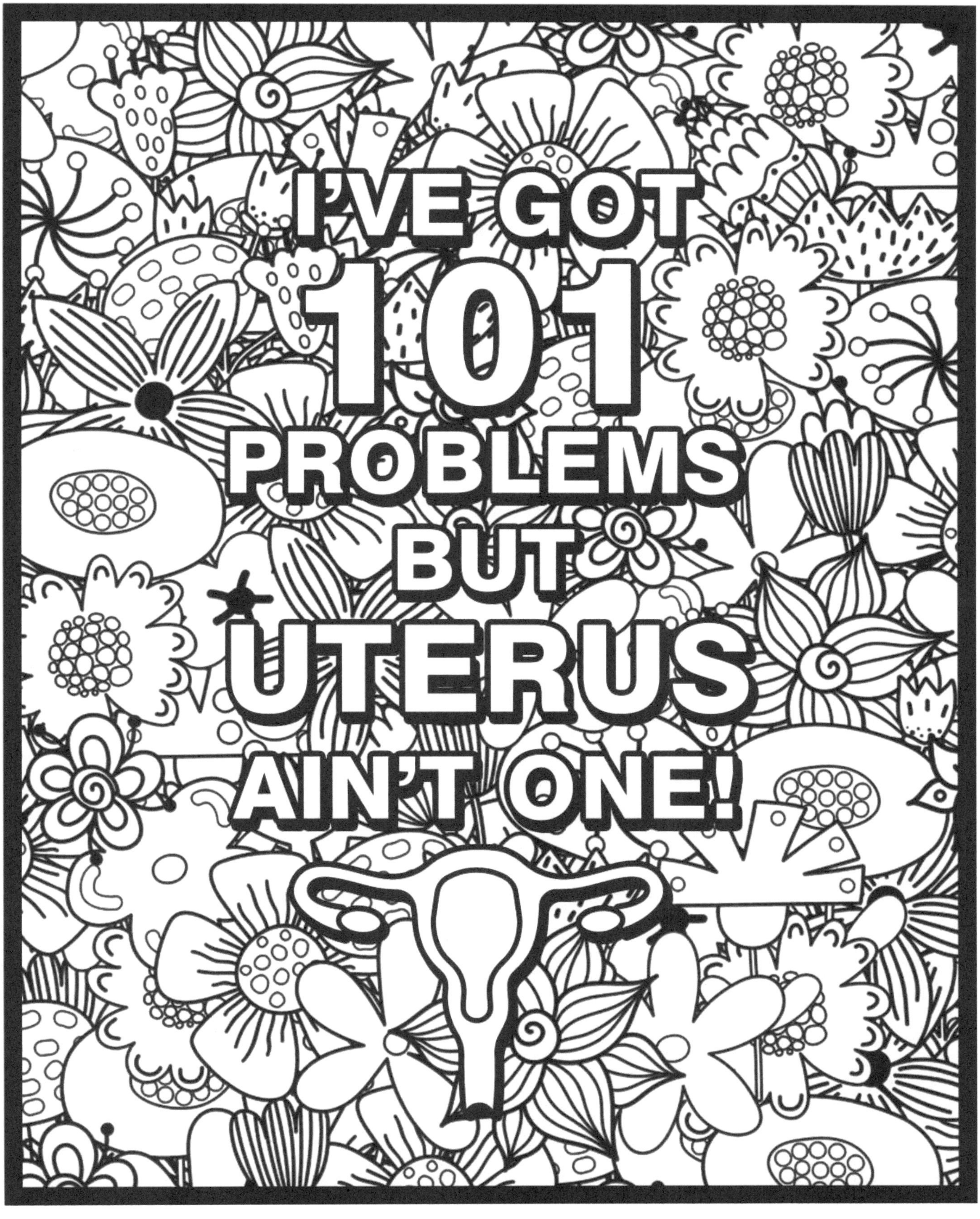
I'VE GOT
101
PROBLEMS
BUT
UTERUS
AIN'T ONE!

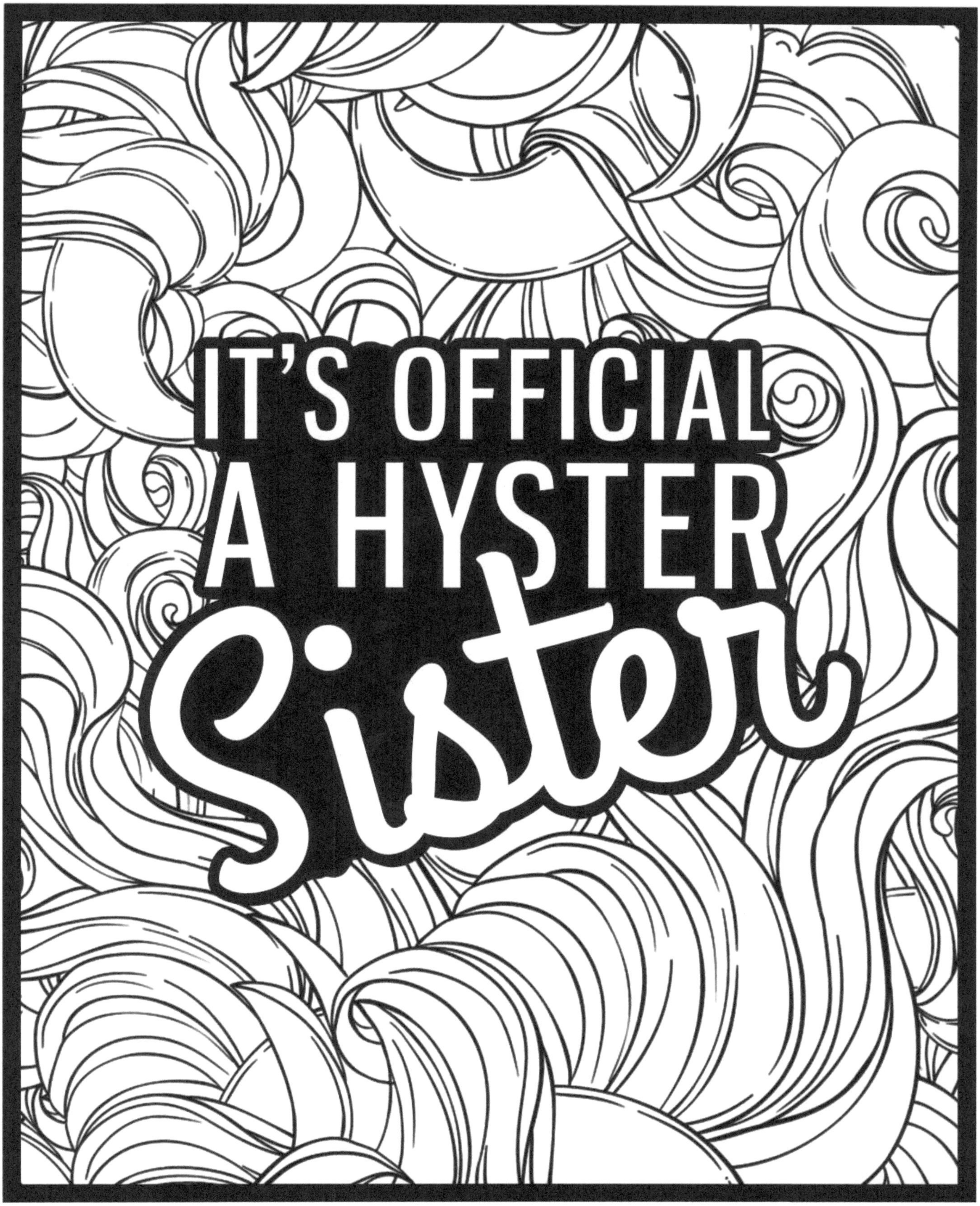
IT'S OFFICIAL
A HYSTER
Sister

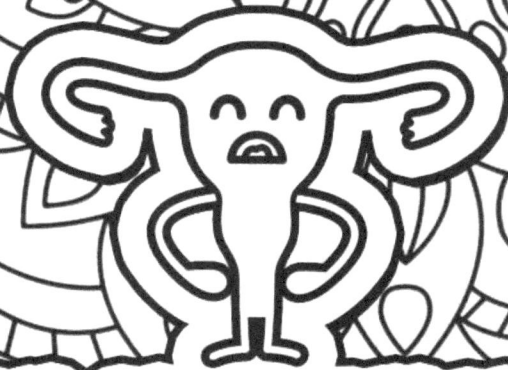

MY UTERUS TRIED TO KILL ME!

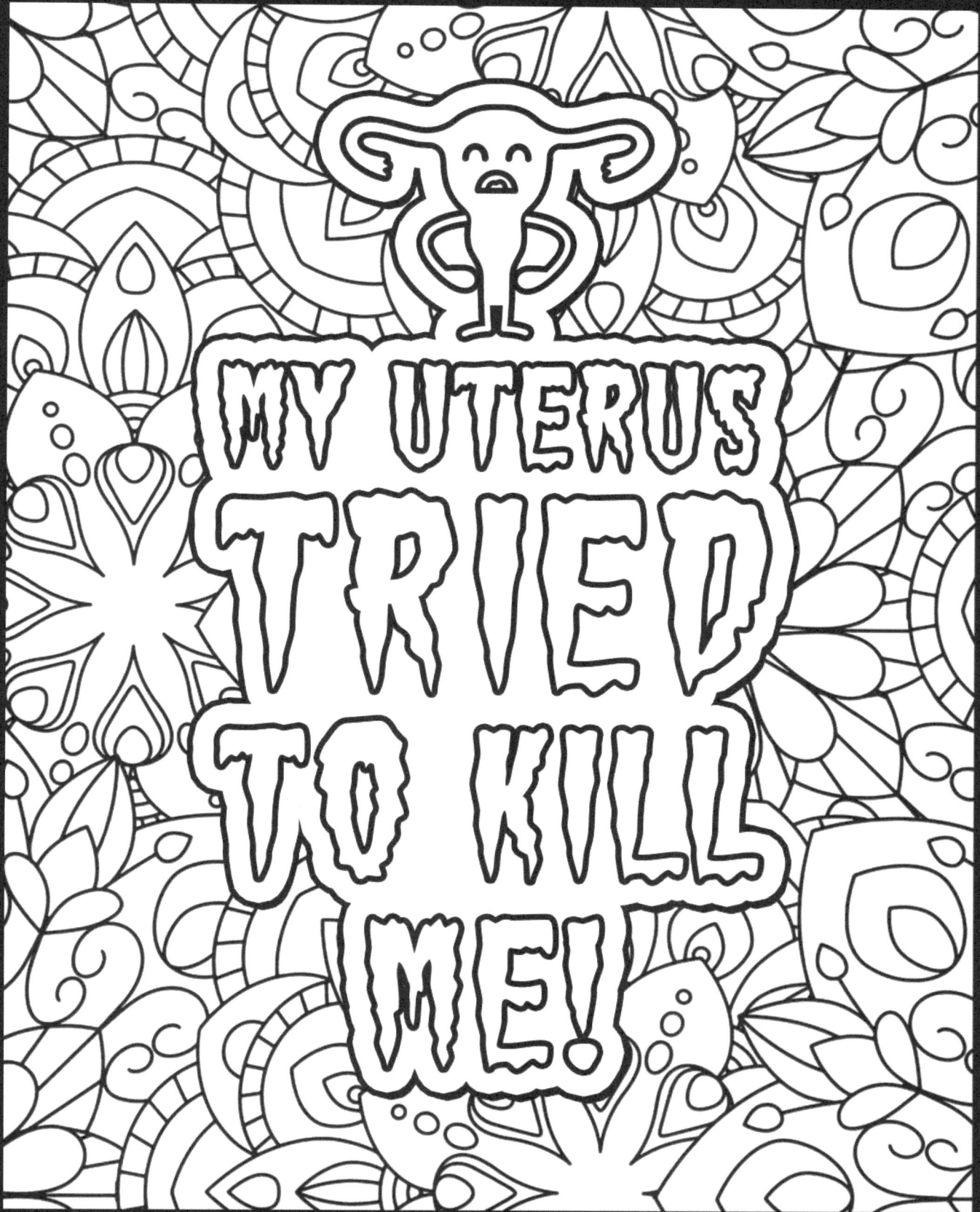

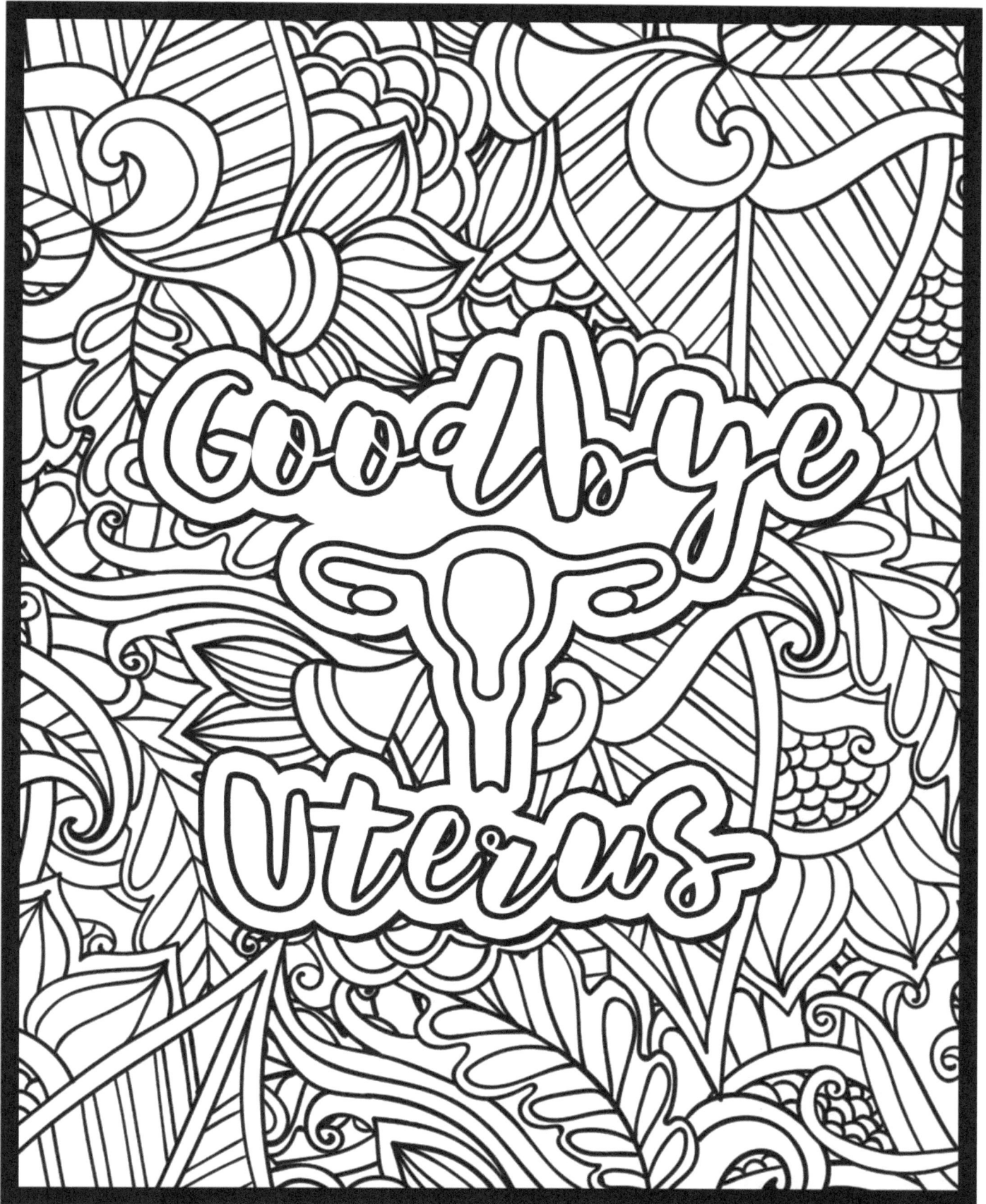
Goodbye Uterus

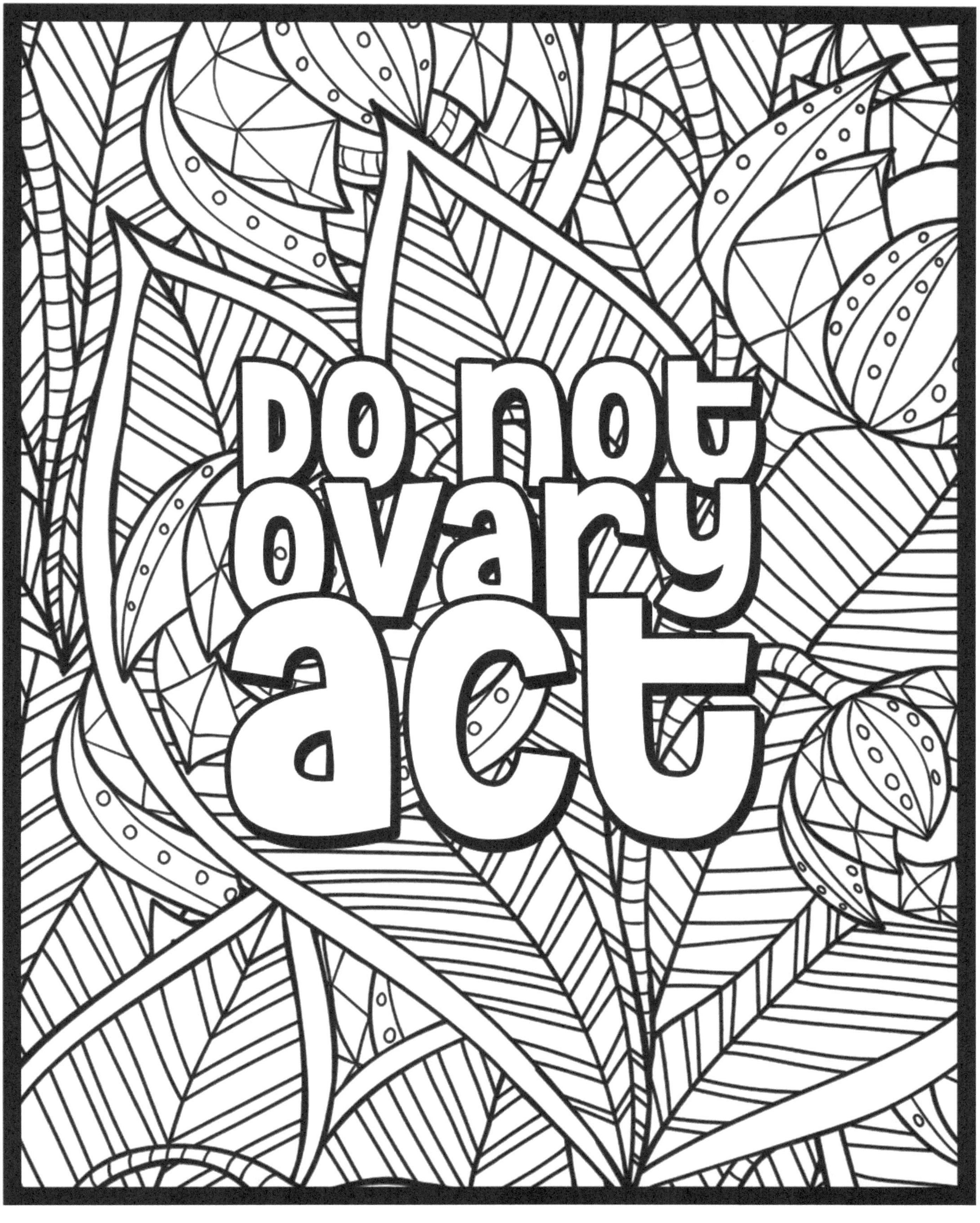
Do not
ovary
act

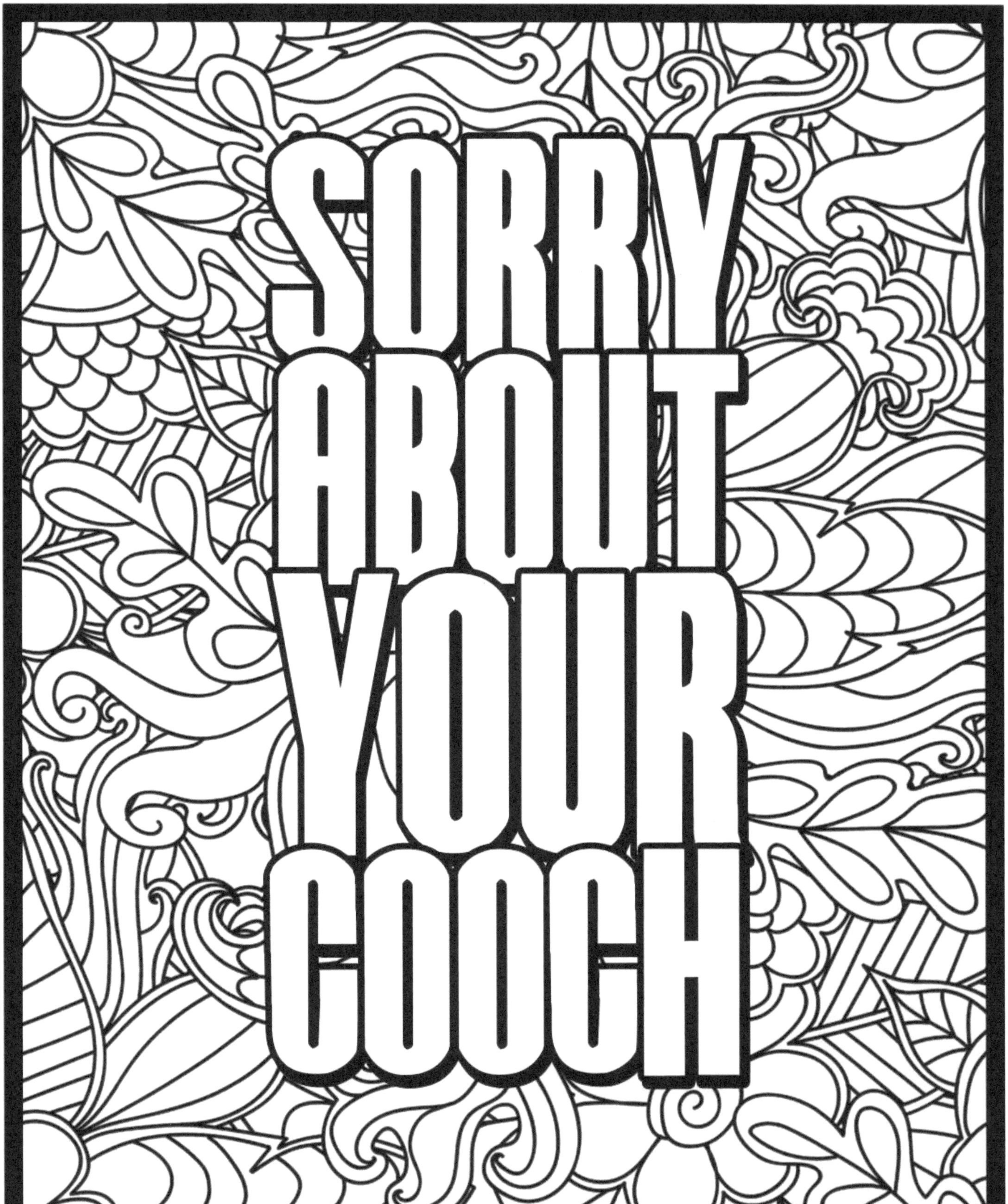
SORRY
ABOUT
YOUR
COOCH

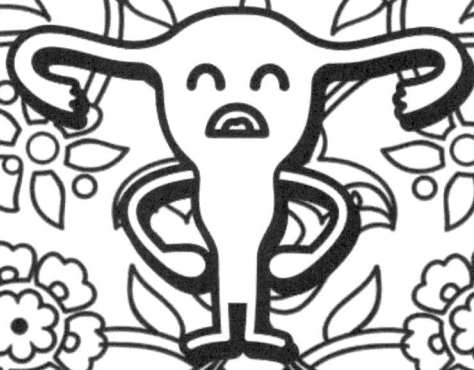

My Uterus and I are breaking up

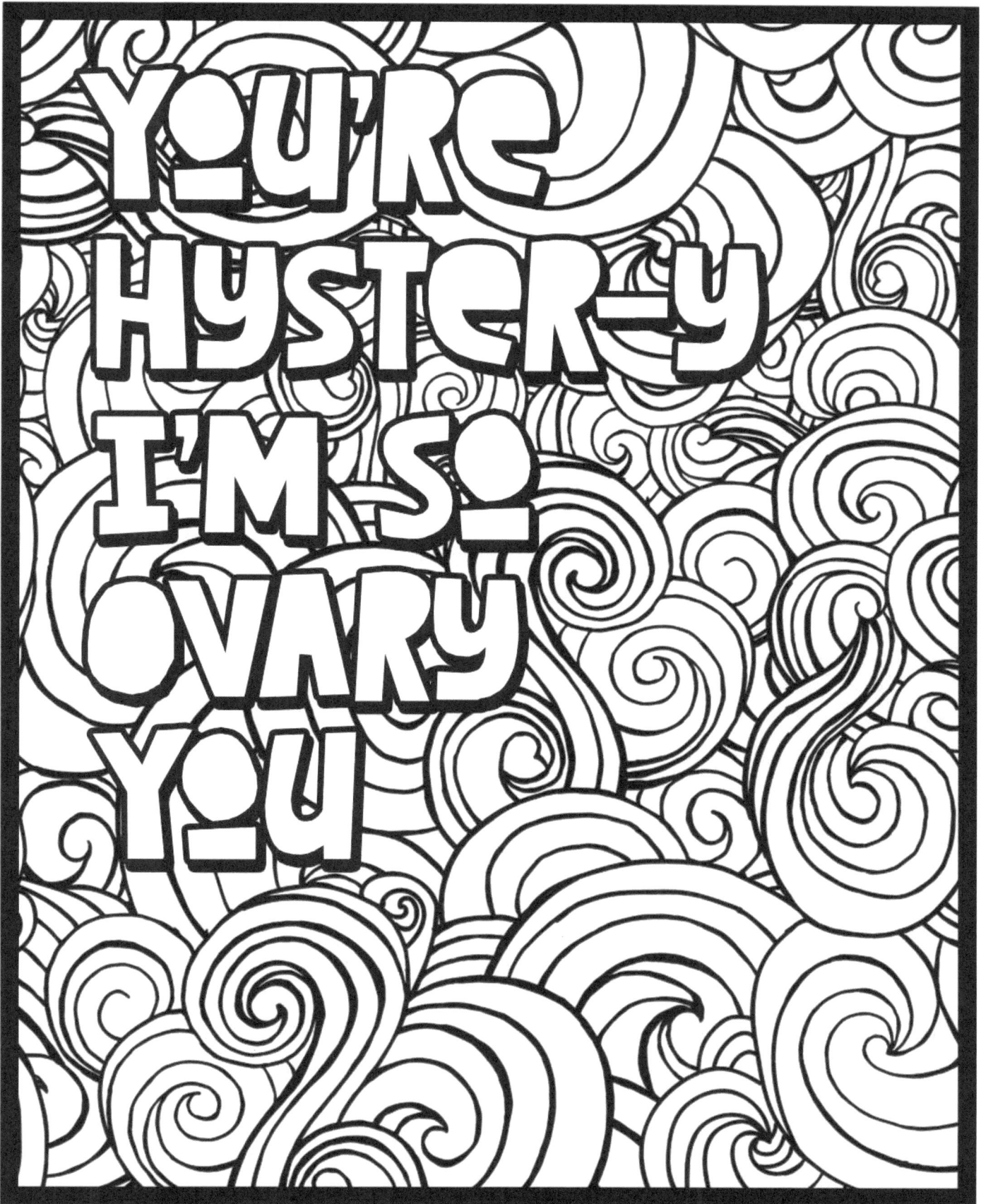

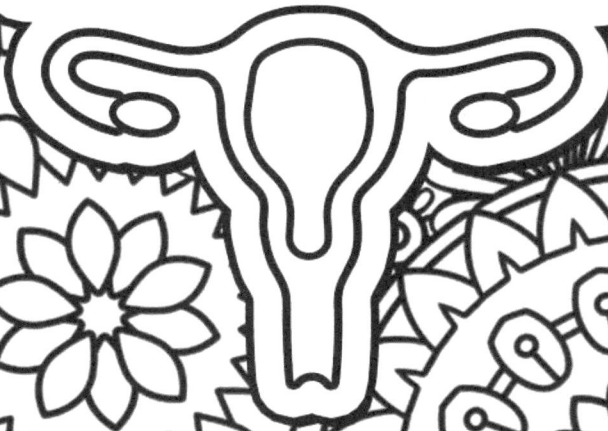

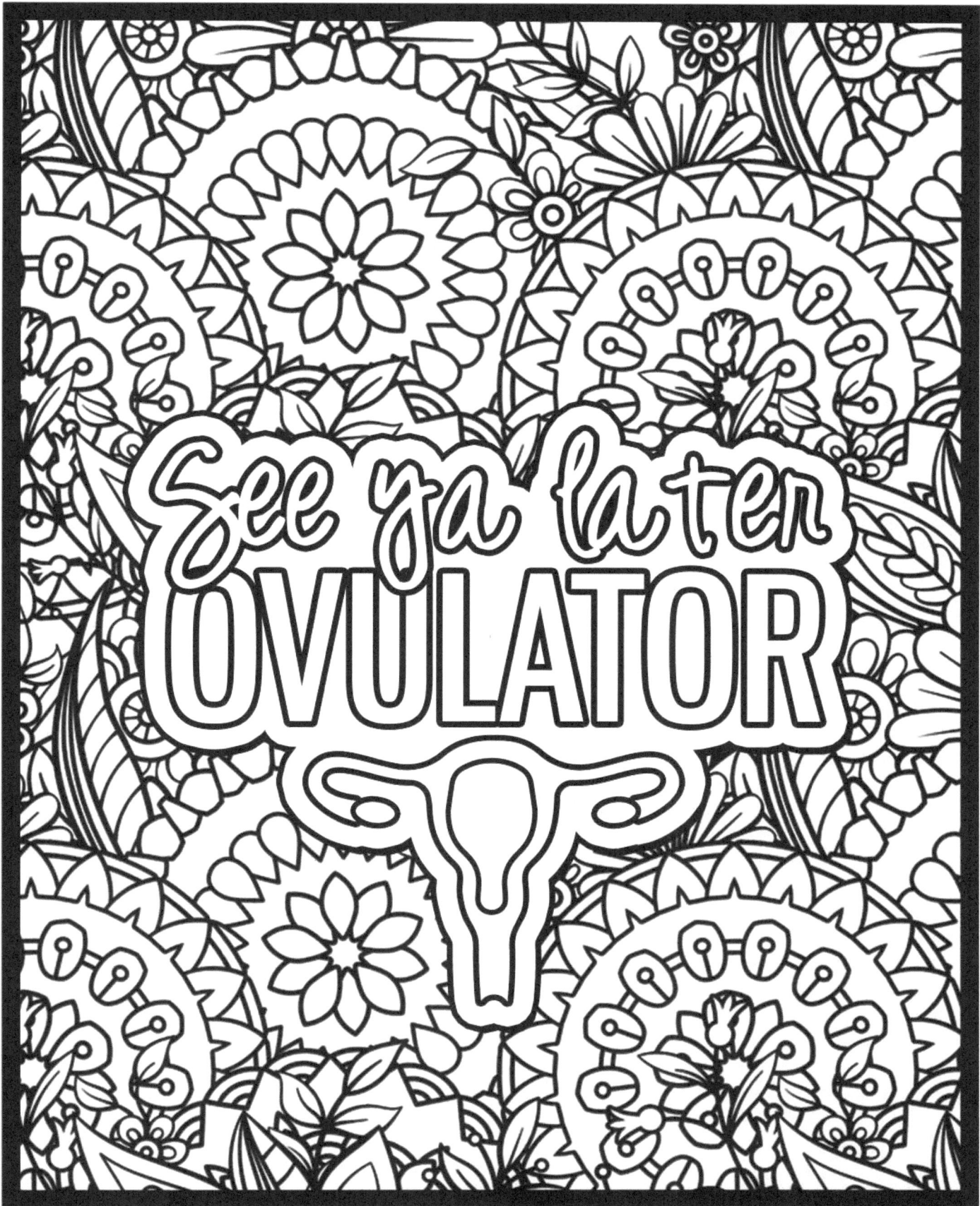

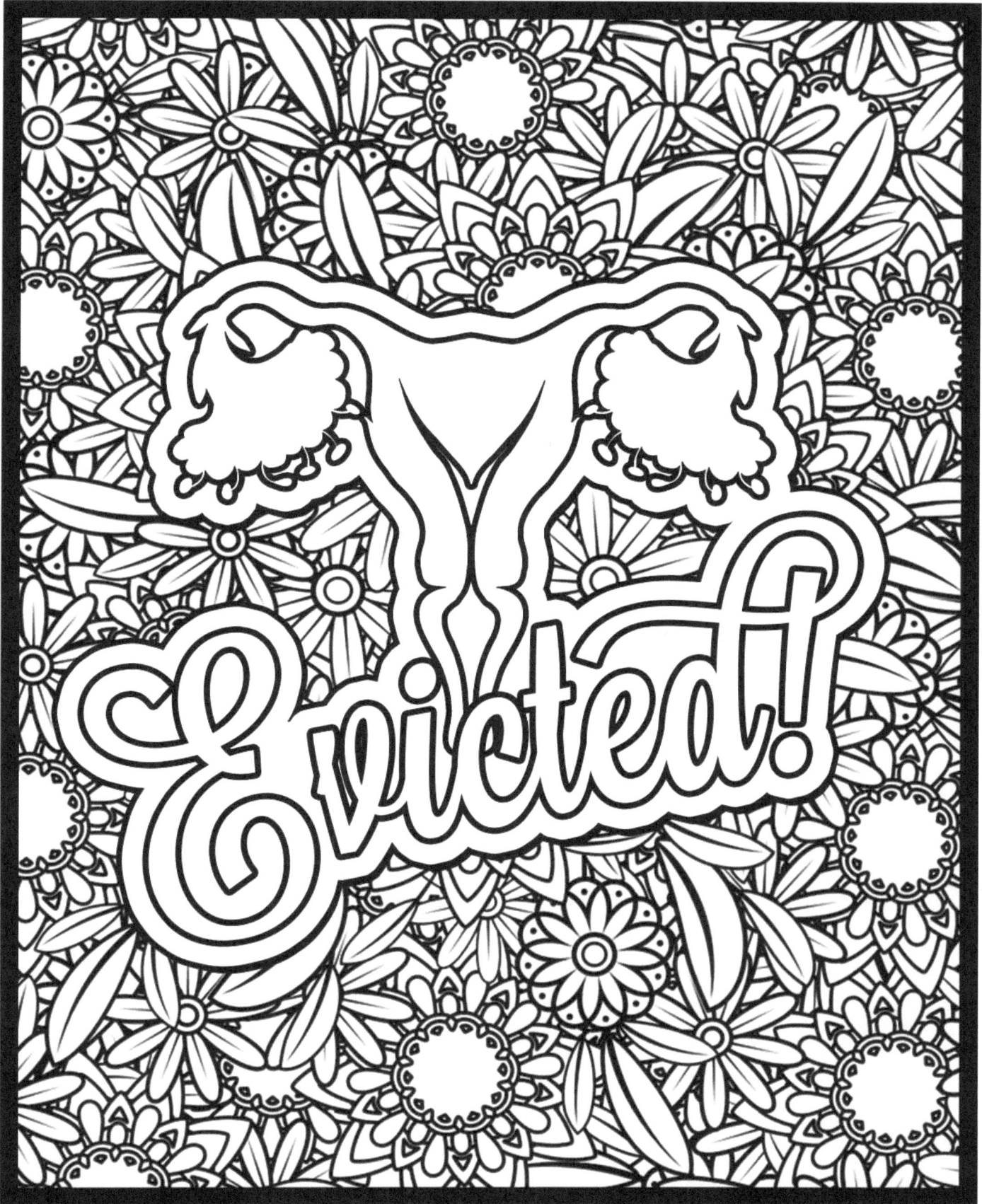

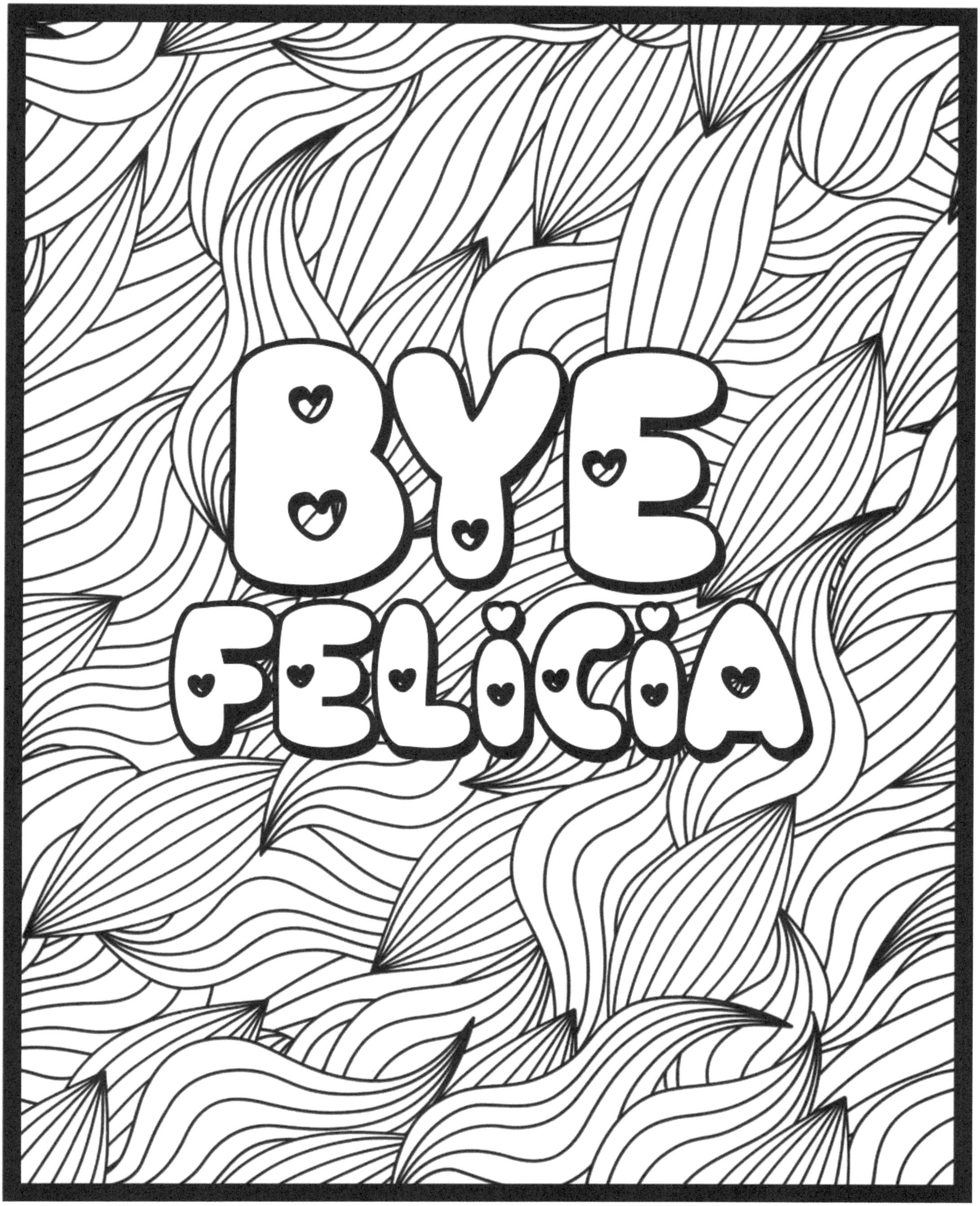
BYE
FELICIA

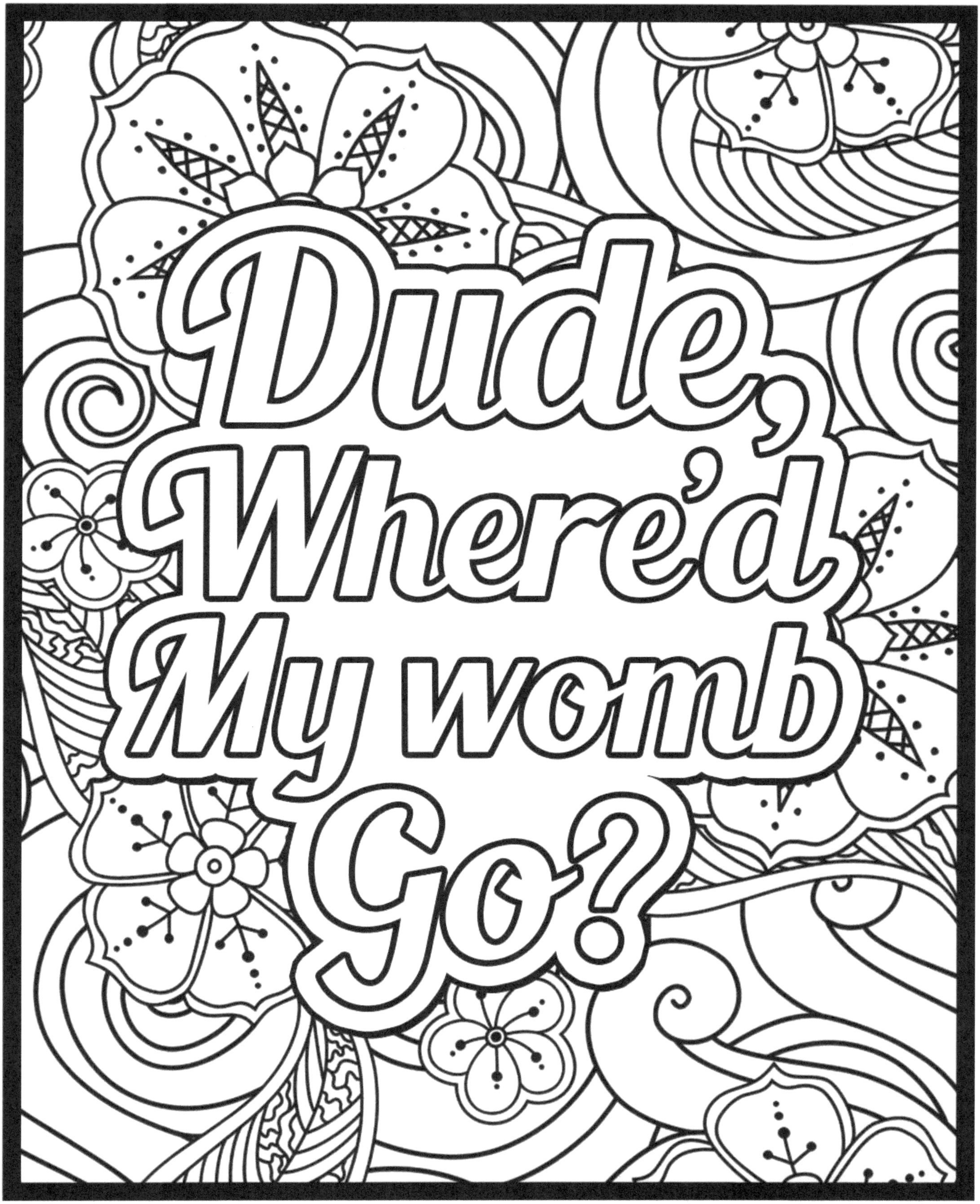
Dude,
Where'd
My womb
Go?

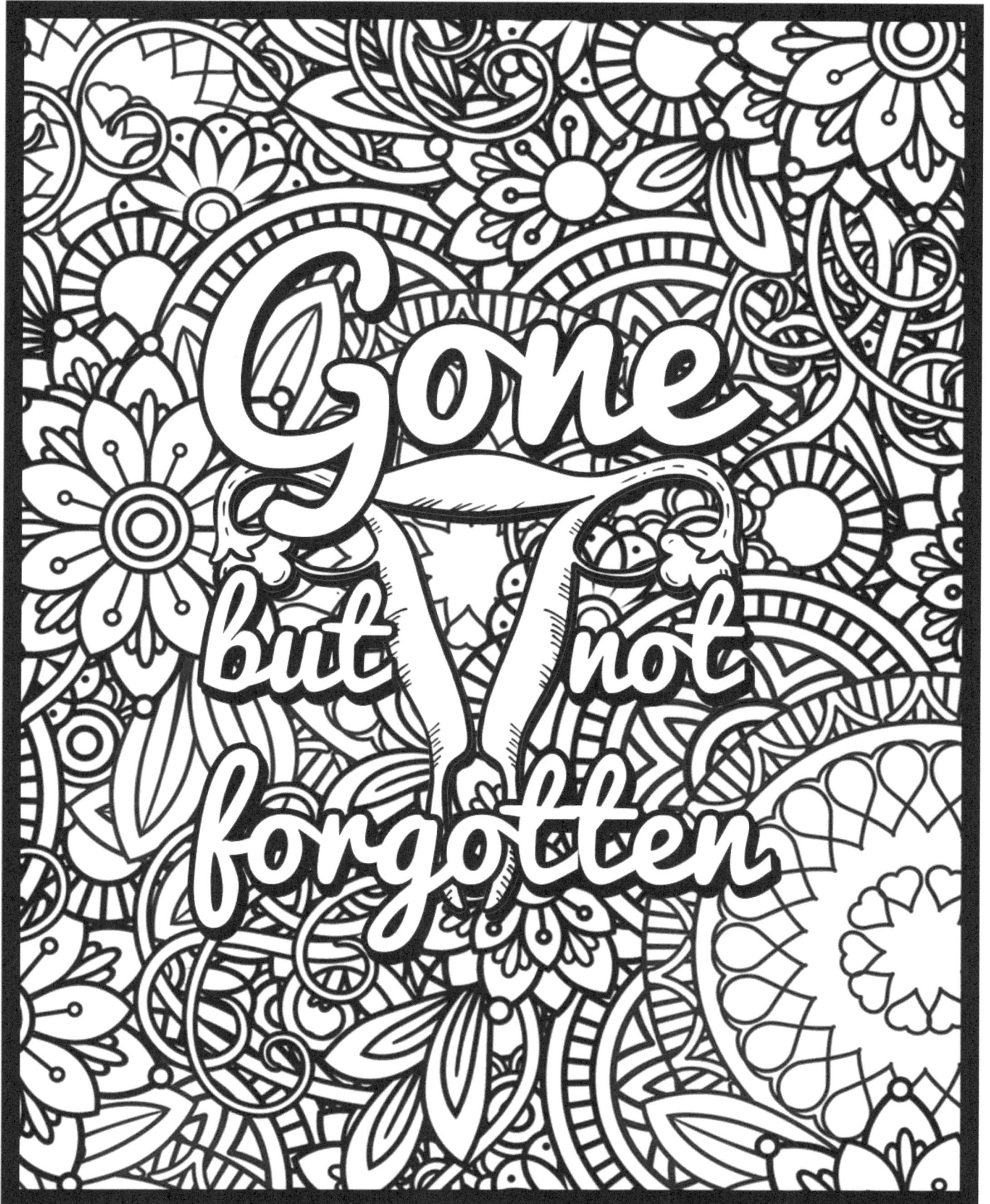

Uterus? Ain't Nobody Got Time For that

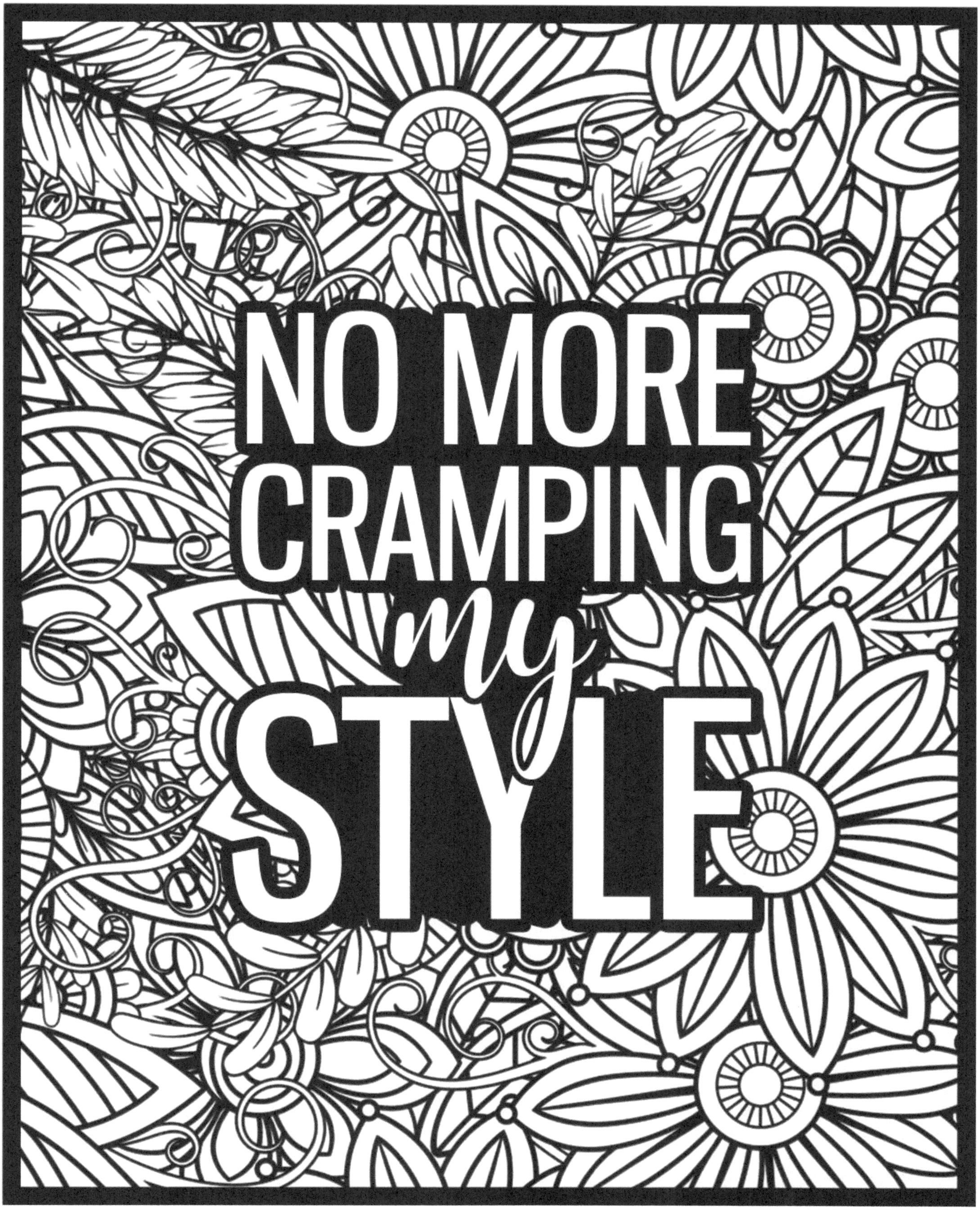
NO MORE
CRAMPING
my
STYLE

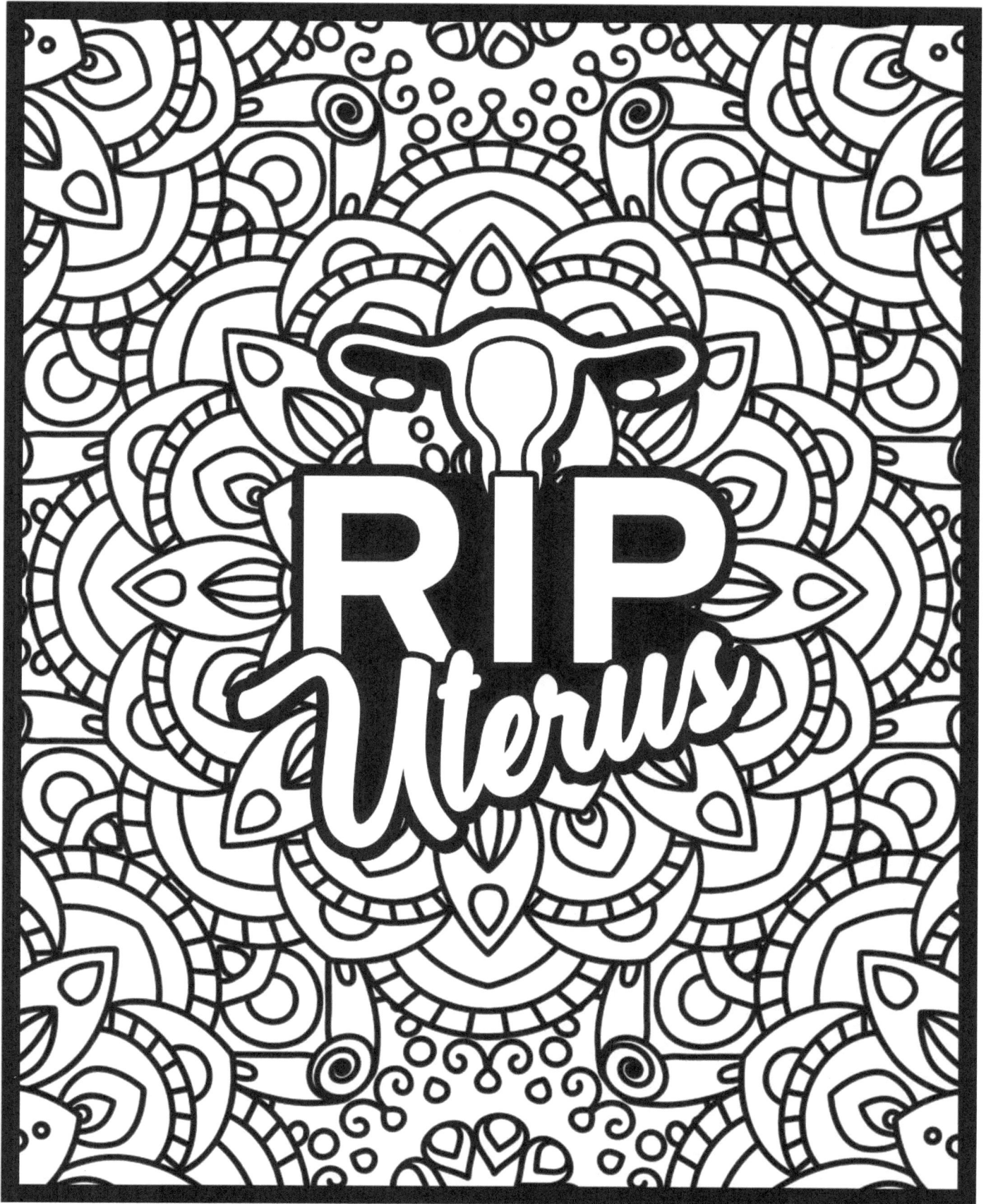

MONTHLY SUBSCRIPTION CANCELLED

STILL AWESOME WITHOUT MY UTERUS